Lyssa Esteves Souto Capuchinho
Cássio de Almeida Lima
Maria A. Vieira

Assessment of the Quality of Life of University Health Teachers

Lyssa Esteves Souto Capuchinho
Cássio de Almeida Lima
Maria A. Vieira

Assessment of the Quality of Life of University Health Teachers

The Context of a Public University

ScienciaScripts

Imprint

Cover image: www.ingimage.com

This book is a translation from the original published under ISBN 978-3-330-77357-8.

Publisher:
Sciencia Scripts
is a trademark of
Dodo Books Indian Ocean Ltd. and OmniScriptum S.R.L publishing group

120 High Road, East Finchley, London, N2 9ED, United Kingdom
Str. Armeneasca 28/1, office 1, Chisinau MD-2012, Republic of Moldova, Europe
Managing Directors: Ieva Konstantinova, Victoria Ursu
info@omniscriptum.com

Printed at: see last page
ISBN: 978-620-8-64790-2

SUMMARY

AUTHORS

Lyssa Esteves Souza Souto[1]

[1]Nurse, graduated from the State University of Montes Claros. Montes Claros, MG, Brazil. Specialist in Teaching in Higher Education at Faculdade Dom Bosco. Curitiba, PR, Brazil.

Càssio de Almeida Lima[2]

[2]Nurse, graduated from the State University of Montes Claros. Specialist in Higher Education Didactics and Methodology. Master's student in the *Stricto Sensu* Postgraduate Program in Health, Society and Environment, Federal University of the Jequitinhonha and Mucuri Valleys. Diamantina, MG, Brazil.

Maria Aparecida Vieira[3]

[3]Nurse, graduated from the Federal University of Minas Gerais. Master's in Nursing from the Federal University of Minas Gerais. PhD in Sciences from the Federal University of São Paulo. Professor in the Nursing Department at the State University of Montes Claros. Professor of the *Stricto Sensu* Postgraduate Program in Primary Health Care at the State University of Montes Claros. Montes Claros, MG, Brazil.

Sarah Martins Souza[4]

[4]Nurse, graduated from the State University of Montes Claros. Montes Claros, MG, Brazil.

Mayara Karoline Silva Lacerda[5]

[5]Nurse, graduated from the State University of Montes Claros. Specialist in Family Health from the State University of Montes Claros. Montes Claros, MG, Brazil.

Fernanda Marques da Costa[6]

[6]Nurse, graduated from the State University of Montes Claros. Master's and Doctorate in Health Sciences from the State University of Montes Claros. Professor in the Nursing Department at the State University of Montes Claros. Professor of the *Stricto Sensu* Postgraduate Program in Primary Health Care at the State University of Montes Claros. Montes Claros, MG, Brazil.

Antônio Prates Caldeira[7]

7Doctor, graduated from the Federal University of Minas Gerais. Master's and PhD in Health Sciences from the Federal University of Minas Gerais. Professor in the Department of Women's and Children's Health at the State University of Montes Claros. Professor of the *Stricto Sensu* Postgraduate Program in Health Sciences at the State University of Montes Claros. Montes Claros, MG, Brazil.

DEDICATORY

To God, who created us and was creative in this task. To my parents, siblings and husband for their encouragement and constant support. And to all the authors who participated with great dedication and spared no effort to complete this book.

ACKNOWLEDGMENTS

To Unimontes, for the grant from the Institutional Scholarship Program for Scientific Initiation (PIBIC).

To the teachers of the undergraduate courses who kindly agreed to take part in this research.

CHAPTER 1

QUALITY OF LIFE: A CONTEXTUALIZATION OF HISTORICAL CONCEPTUAL ASPECTS AND RELATIONSHIPS WITH HEALTH

The expression quality of life has its roots in both Eastern and Western culture. It is found in ancient Chinese philosophy, related to areas such as art, literature, philosophy, traditional medicine, the positive and negative forces represented by the concepts of Yin and Yang, which, according to this philosophy, establish that quality of life can be achieved when Yin and Yang are balanced. It is also related to the Aristotelian view, according to which happiness, one of the axes inherent to quality of life, can be defined as a certain type of virtuous activity of the soul, capable of providing fullness and fulfillment (ZHAN, 1992).

According to Beck, Budó and Gonzales (1999), the term quality of life appeared before Aristotle, associated with values such as happiness and virtue, which, when obtained, would provide human beings with a good life. It was also linked to expressions such as well-being, aspiration, need and satisfaction. It was referenced in 1947 by the World Health Organization (WHO) as a concept of health, covering, among other things, standards of living, housing, working conditions and access to health services.

This expression began to be used in the United States after World War II as a synonym for the acquisition of material goods such as houses, cars, investments, money and travel. Later, its concept was expanded to measure the economic development of a society, by comparing different cities and regions using economic indicators such as gross domestic product (GDP) and per capita income. At another time, it began to measure social development by parameters linked to health, education, housing and transportation. In contemporary society, the subject of quality of life has been widely discussed. It is receiving increasing attention, not only in scientific literature, but also in the media - especially in advertising and political campaigns; and it is also considered a powerful term in popular discourse and often even becomes a cliché

(FARQUHAR, 1995; BOWLING, 1997).

It began to be used in the United States of America shortly after the Second World War to show the material goods acquired in the post-war period, such as travel and investments. Subsequently, the concept expanded to encompass the great economic development of various localities through economic indicators such as gross domestic product and per capita income. Over time, it also began to incorporate the social concept and to measure development through other indicators, such as housing, health and education (ARRONQUI *et al.*, 2011).

According to Paschoal (2001), the concept of quality of life has expanded over time, encompassing socio-economic and human development, or the objective aspect, and individual perception, or the subjective aspect, and the perception of quality of life changes from person to person and is dynamic in each one (CARR; GIBSON; ROBSON, 2001). Due to its subjectivity, complexity and multidimensionality, it is difficult to define quality of life, as it depends on intrinsic and extrinsic characteristics that influence each person's individual concept (ROCHA; FELLI, 2004) and involves aspects of family, social, environmental, cultural, comfort and well-being (MINAYO; HARTZ; BUSS, 2000).

In a holistic context, quality of life is defined by Ravagnani, Domingos and Miyazaki (2007) as an individual's perception of their position in life, in the context of the culture and value system in which they live and in relation to their goals, expectations, standards and concerns. It encompasses psychological conditions and well-being, social interactions, economic, vocational, religious and spiritual factors. For Panzini *et al.* (2007) the more recent theme of quality of life encompasses and transcends the field of health, since it involves other dimensions. The quality of life construct is broad, multidimensional and transdisciplinary.

Quality of life is an eminently human notion, which comes close to the levels of satisfaction found in family, love, social and environmental life and in the existential aesthetic itself. It presupposes the ability to make a cultural synthesis of all the subsidies that a given society considers to be its standards of comfort and well-being.

The term has many meanings, reflecting the knowledge, experiences and values of individuals and collectivities who refer to it in different times, spaces and contexts, and is a social construction under the aegis of cultural relativity. It can be said that the issue of quality of life concerns the standards that society itself sets and mobilizes to achieve, consciously or unconsciously, positive changes in living conditions and lifestyles, assigning a significant portion of responsibility to the field of health. As far as health is concerned, theoretical notions come together as a social result of the collective construction of standards of comfort that a given society establishes as parameters for its members. In this sense, the notion of quality of life moves through a polysemic semantic field in which conditions and lifestyles are linked; the arguments of sustainable development and human ecology; the fields of democracy, development and human and social rights (CASTELLANOS, 1997; MINAYO; HARTZ; BUSS, 2000).

According to Panzini *et al.* (2007), quality of life is also considered a polysemic term, with a tendency to value people's personal appreciation of their life and well-being. As such, it is influenced by individual and family history, by expectations, but also by the media and mass advertising. It is a recent concept, which encompasses and transcends the concept of health, and is made up of various domains or dimensions, such as physical, psychological and environmental. Explanations of quality of life originate from different approaches, which can be objective, in which the degree of satisfaction of basic human needs and the needs created as a result of the level of socio-economic development of a given society predominates; or they can be subjective, in which the state of well-being, happiness, love and personal fulfillment is analyzed (OLIVEIRA; CIAMPONE, 2008).

Nowadays, the term quality of life has a concept that involves parameters from the areas of health, architecture, urbanism, leisure, gastronomy, sports, education, the environment, public and private security, entertainment, new technologies and everything related to human beings, their culture and their environment. It has expanded over time to encompass socio-economic and human development, objective/subjective aspects and individual perception. The understanding of quality of life changes from person to person and is dynamic in each subjective perception of the process of production, circulation and consumption of goods and wealth (ALMEIDA; GUTIERREZ; MARQUES, 2012).

According to Minayo, Hartz and Buss (2000), there are three eminently sociological aspects that directly influence the organization of quality of life standards. In the first aspect, which is more historical, at a given moment in its socio-economic evolution, a specific society has a different quality of life standard to the same society at another historical stage. The second aspect is cultural, based on values and needs that are constructed and hierarchized differently by peoples. The third aspect refers to stratification or social classes. In societies where inequalities and heterogeneities are very present, it is clear that standards and conceptions of well-being are also stratified, as the idea of quality of life is linked to the comfort of the upper classes. Cultural relativism, however, does not make it impossible to perceive that a hegemonic model is expanding. This is the model advocated by the Western world, which is urbanized, wealthy and polarized by values that include comfort, pleasure, good food, fashion, household utilities, travel, various material goods, the use of technologies that reduce manual labour, the consumption of art and culture, among other amenities.

In this context, Fiedler (2008) emphasizes that the individual is obliged to meet the demands of contemporaneity, while transforming their behavior in search of greater productivity, greater knowledge, greater scope in their actions, in short, sacrificing themselves in the search for the excellence demanded by their environment. Such pragmatic behavior has consequences, as it interferes with their emotional balance and their quality of life. The increase in competitiveness, the desire to know more and have more, generates a contingent of guilty people, overloaded and under pressure, who end up forgetting the basic values of good coexistence. Xavier (2011) adds that the changes in the world of work are multifaceted and can be summed up in a few general factors, such as consumption and individualism as hegemonic values, the commodification of the world and people, the acceleration of activities and the growing superfluity of work and workers. These factors culminate in the weakening of work as a source of meaning and the alienation of professionals.

It is also a subject that has been consolidated as an important variable in clinical practice and in the production of knowledge in the health field. Its application can result in changes in health care practices and the implementation of new paradigms of the health-disease process based on health promotion, whose socioeconomic, cultural and psychological aspects must be recognized and linked to quality of life, a construct that is thus characterized as eminently interdisciplinary (SEIDL; ZANNON, 2004).

Since the 1980s, this topic has been researched using objective and subjective approaches. The former refers to the degree to which needs are met, depending on their socio-economic expansion, and the latter concerns the person's well-being and their perception of the level of personal fulfillment in the individual and collective spheres (PETRINI, 2013).

Oliveira, Mininel and Felli (2011) point out that, because it is directly linked to aspects of health, the term quality of life is often used as a synonym for health. Despite the obvious relationship between the two conditions, to say that quality of life is having health is to reduce it to a single fragment of all the meanings of the health-disease process, which encompasses countless dimensions of human life. Minayo, Hartz and Buss (2000) add that it has become common in the health sector to repeat the phrase: "health is not illness, health is quality of life". However correct this statement may be, it is usually devoid of meaning and often exposes the difficulty of finding some theoretical and epistemological sense outside the biologicist model that still dominates reflection and practice in the field of public health. It must be pointed out that, although it is known that the state of health of individuals and collectivities, as well as the health system, influences and is influenced by the global environment, it must be recognized that not every aspect of human life is fundamentally a medical or health issue. Thus, stating that the concept of health is related to or should be closer to the notion of quality of life, that health is not merely the absence of disease, expresses dissatisfaction with biomedical reductionism, but does not strengthen reflection.

The minimum and global material level for considering quality of life concerns the satisfaction of the most basic human needs, i.e. food, access to drinking water, housing, education, working conditions, money, information, the environment, health services, leisure and means of transportation. These are material supports referenced by notions of comfort, well-being and individual and collective fulfillment. In today's Western world, it can also be said that unemployment, social exclusion and violence are objectively recognized as the opposite of quality of life. In this way, they are characterized as components that can be measured and compared, even though they must be constantly relativized socially and culturally in different contexts (MINAYO; HARTZ; BUSS, 2000; PENTEADO; PEREIRA, 2007).

Camponogara, Kirchhof and Ramos (2008) explain that relating the concept of quality of life to the current context of vertiginous social changes is necessary in order to interpret the agents that interfere with the population's morbidity and mortality patterns. For a long time, the concept of quality of life was related to the supposed positive effects of technical-scientific progress, with a consequent lack of reflection on its harmful effects. However, it is believed that the health sector is undergoing a process of immersion, reflexivity and re-evaluation of its epistemological foundations, with emphasis on valuing people's subjectivity, with greater autonomy over the health-disease process and the search for their quality of life. Quality of life implies considering assumptions that have repercussions on theoretical conceptions and social practices that are open to multidimensionality, that recognize the subjectivity of individuals, that attribute centrality to the determinants of the health-disease process and enable a new look at health praxis. The concept of quality of life has long been part of discussions in the field of health and various conceptual approaches have underpinned actions to improve humanity's quality of life.

Minayo, Hartz and Buss (2000) analyse that the discourse on the relationship between health and quality of life, although unspecific and generalizing, has existed since the birth of social medicine in the 18th and 19th centuries, when systematic research began to highlight the importance of quality of life and offer support for public policies and social movements. Panzini *et al.* (2007) add that the introduction of the concept of quality of life as a measure of health outcomes came about in the 1970s, at a time of progress in the field of medicine. This progress led to longer life expectancy, as previously lethal diseases, such as infections, became curable or at least had their symptoms controlled or their normal course slowed down. This extension has come at the cost of living with milder or asymptomatic forms of the diseases, making it important to have ways of understanding how people have lived these extra years.

From a more focused perspective, quality of life in health is centered on the ability to live without illness or to overcome the difficulties of conditions or states of morbidity. This is due to the fact that, in general, professionals work in areas where they can have a direct influence, i.e. they try to alleviate pain, discomfort and illness, to intervene in problems that often lead to dependency and discomfort, either to avoid them or to minimize the consequences of them or of the interventions carried out to diagnose or treat them. The subject of quality of life is dealt with from many different perspectives, whether from science, common sense, objective or subjective analysis, or in individual or collective approaches. In health, when seen in a holistic sense, it is based on an understanding of fundamental human needs, both material and spiritual, and has its most relevant basis in the concept of health promotion (MINAYO; HARTZ; BUSS, 2000).

It is known that poor quality of life interferes with the physical and mental health of workers, influences the planning and performance of activities, and can be associated with stress, nervous tension, muscle fatigue, repetitive strain injuries and work-related musculoskeletal disorders (DAVILA; CASAGRANDE; PEREIRA, 2010).

CHAPTER 2

QUALITY OF LIFE IN THE WORKING CONTEXT OF UNIVERSITY HEALTH TEACHERS

The object of work in the health sector is the individual and/or collective human body involved in the health-disease process. The means and instruments applied are knowledge, diagnostic equipment and the workforce, including forms of organization, division and relationships. The work relationships of the professionals who work in this area differ in parallel with the work process carried out. The same is true of teaching, where teaching is seen as an intellectual dynamic and is therefore more privileged than caring, because conditions such as working hours, working conditions and salaries are more favorable (ROCHA; FELLI, 2004).

Teachers in the health sector play an important role as agents of health, considering that they do not only communicate knowledge, but are also agents of transformation who possess singularities in their knowledge. His practice has an effect on the training of new professionals, as he becomes an important vector in the subjectivation processes of the subject for professional and personal training, making this profession a highly enriching activity that provides various skills linked to the field of health. In order to satisfy the population, it is essential that both teachers and academics understand the meaning of quality of life and the value it has for the subjects with whom they interact on a daily basis, since the way and the amount of processing of their activities will provide or not the quality of life of these educators (GARCIA; OLIVEIRA; BARROS, 2008).

Koifman (2011) emphasizes that the university plays a decisive role in the training of professionals, not only because it demonstrates resolubility in comparison with other institutions, but also because of its unique role in defining the ethics of national development and because it is a special locus for social criticism and transformation. Perceiving university institutions as instances that foster debates cultural means understanding them as the driving force behind procedures for the creation, appropriation and transmission of knowledge, values and representations that come together at a level of the educational system defined as superior by any society. One of the dimensions of national needs focuses above all on the training of health professionals guided by the future direction of science, and only the university can fully contemplate this.

Garcia, Oliveira and Barros (2008) point out that teachers are subjected to long working hours and demand an intense and complex cognitive component with the use of multiple codes and diversification of activities, requiring rapid decision-making. Teachers' work is subjugated to an organizational prototype that is generally theoretically geared towards the rudiments of humanity. Situations persist that de-characterize the educational system, understood as an essential factor in the manufacture of powerful ways of life. They are often based on exacerbated competition, productivism and loyalty to market interests.

According to Conceiçao *et al.* (2012), the constant responsibilities of teachers linked to the teaching-learning process in health, which includes the academic and the population, as well as the associated ethical issues, are constantly limiting quality of life and causing health problems when they are not addressed. This problem is even more significant because of the work overload imposed by academic activities, where educators are obliged to take their work outside the workplace.

According to Ramos *et al.* (2011), the obstacles experienced by teachers in the daily life of universities are linked to the transformations articulated with science, education and work. The teaching staff feel encouraged to reflect on their daily practices in the academic space and in the health services, but they also experience difficulties in consolidating proposals for change and drawing up consistent plans.

Teachers find it difficult to reconcile spaces for interaction with people in the teaching-learning process, with a view to promoting a pleasant collective environment, even in situations of conflict, while at the same time developing self-care strategies (CONCEIÇÂO *et al.*, 2012). They make excessive demands of themselves, are leaders, opinion formers, and play an important role in training students and guiding scientific activities. Stress is present in their work, along with competition, advisory services, consultancies, excessive assignments in undergraduate and postgraduate courses and short deadlines (CARAN *et al.*, 2011).

There are countless negative experiences that revive a discourse of permanent tension between teacher and student: offensive statements, belittling teachers and their work, comparisons between professionals and inappropriate ways of relating in the academic environment (RAMOS *et al.*, 2011).

In a study by Xavier (2011), carried out in various Spanish cities between 2008 and 2009, with the aim of providing a preliminary comparative and qualitative mapping of the themes related to labor changes within organizational capitalism that appear in workers' fantasies and dreams, it was identified that university professors wanted to have more autonomy in the institution, to be a good professional and to improve their training. Not being listened to, not knowing the academics and not being prepared were situations that differed from those desired. The chronic acceleration of work, the lack of time, the small number of teachers for a large number of students can lead to emotional detachment or alienation from the act of teaching undergraduates. The more experienced teachers showed that feelings of anguish and unpreparedness contrasted with the way they saw themselves and their work. The conflict between the desire to offer quality teaching and, at the same time, dedicate themselves to research and bureaucratic tasks; the work situation of a heavy workload and the desire for professional advancement; the need for recognition and an organizational climate marked by constant demands and disagreements with management, were reported by the professors.

According to Martinez, Vitta and Lopes (2009), the more time teachers devote to their work, the less time they have available for everyday activities, such as household chores, family care, health and leisure, resulting in an overload of personal and family demands and an affected quality of life. It is not possible to carry out your professional work or any other activity constantly, because you need breaks for rest, distraction, sleep, so as not to become irritated or tired.

Teachers are undervalued, which makes personal, social and professional investment impossible. Most of them work in unhealthy places, in poorly ventilated classrooms, with noise, dust and chalk, as well as indiscipline and disrespect from students (PENTEADO; PEREIRA, 2007). In view of this, teacher dissatisfaction is constant in the educational environment, which has countless consequences for the quality of interpersonal relationships in the workplace. Often, these relationships are not in line with the expectations and representations of educators and affect their own personal fulfillment. Unhealthy competition, political influence in the workplace, aggressive behavior among colleagues and academics are among the stressors at work. These agents contribute to the occurrence of conflicts of values, when there is disharmony between the teacher's personal principles and the demands of the job (MULATO; BUENO; FRANCO, 2010).

According to Santos, Cavalcante and Berardinelli (2010), personal life is experienced in parallel with professional activities, the remuneration received, the institutional environment, relationships of power and with bosses and colleagues, as well as the need to meet the need to socialize with family and friends and these factors can be the reason for satisfaction or not with the work developed.

Martinez, Vitta and Lopes (2009) point out that professors are a group of workers who live with the presence of various psychosocial risk factors on a daily basis. Generally, their working hours are long and, if they belong to a university, the multiple demands involve carrying out research, obtaining funding for studies, career growth and mentoring undergraduates.

Competition for positions and publications and the educational context can generate stress for everyone involved. The continuous exposure of workers to psychosocial occupational risks can lead to the emergence of mental and behavioral disorders, resulting not from isolated factors, but from work contexts in interaction with the body and psychic apparatus of workers. The actions involved in the act of working can produce biological dysfunctions and injuries, psychic reactions to pathogenic work situations and trigger psychopathological processes (BRASIL, 2001).

In a study by Caran *et al.* (2011), carried out in a public higher education institution in the interior of the state of Sao Paulo in 2006, the aim was to investigate the existence of psychosocial occupational risks (POR) in the work environment of university professors and the repercussions on their health, it was identified that the main agents of psychosocial risks and their repercussions on workers' health were overload, especially mental overload, stress, pressure, conflicting interpersonal relationships and lack of planning. These risks influence teachers' health and cause stress, anxiety, insomnia/sleep difficulties, headaches, gastritis, bad mood, irritability, tiredness and fatigue.

Santos, Cavalcante and Berardinelli (2010) add that negative feelings, such as anxiety and depression, are part of the daily lives of the vast majority of teachers and cause difficulties in their work. This reality is due to the complexity of the theory-learning-practice fit and the demands arising from scientific and technological advances in the health area. According to Ferreira *et al.* (2009), hierarchy and the lack of autonomy for teachers are components that generate suffering. The pressure and precarious working conditions contribute to professional burnout, reduced work performance, ageing and the manifestation of certain somatic illnesses.

Gampel, Karsch and Ferreira (2010) state that teachers rely on their voice as one of their main working tools and use it for long periods of time. Because of this, they are prone to acquiring vocal problems, as their busy routines and excessive workload mean that a significant proportion of them do not notice signs that indicate vocal alterations. However, they do not identify the relationship between their voice and emotions that can influence their social life, because they consider vocal problems to be inherent to their profession. The worsening of these problems can compromise their well-being, as some of these professionals tend to take time off work because of voice problems, which can lead to emotional, economic and social problems.

Garcia, Oliveira and Barros (2008) emphasize that producing alternatives for prevention and health promotion in the workplace makes work an active agent. Teachers themselves are able to look for strategies to improve their quality of life by recovering the social function of pleasure and solidarity in work relationships, through the external and internal changes they seek.

Silvério *et al.* (2010) point out that data from the literature provides a paradoxical image of the teaching work environment, in which there is simultaneously a powerful space for human interactions, meetings, exchanges of knowledge, experiences, feelings and energies, which help to promote teachers' quality of life, but which is also a place subject to conflicts of various kinds, which can cause constant situations of stress and limitations to integral health.

In view of the above, it can be seen that there are countless situations which do not promote quality of life in the course of teaching in the health area. Based on this assumption, the idea of researching quality of life in the university environment is mobilized by everyday teaching practices (SILVÉRIO *et al.*, 2010), justifying the preparation of this study, which contains the following guiding question:

- *"What is the assessment of teachers in undergraduate health courses at a public university of their quality of life?"* For this purpose, we opted for the definition of quality of life proposed by the World Health Organization (WHO), where there is a working team that studies quality of life issues linked to health. The group, called WHOQOL GROUP (World Health Organization Quality of Life Group), considers that the definition of quality of life must take into account the individual's perception and their relationship with the environment. It defines quality of life as an individual's perception of their position in life, within the framework of their culture and value system and in relation to their goals, expectations, standards and concerns. It is a wide-ranging concept affected in a complex way by physical health, psychological state, level of independence, social relationships and relationships with the characteristics of the individual's environment (WHOQOL 1994; FLECK *et al.*, 2000).

According to Terra, Secco and Robazzi (2011), weighing up aspects of work activity and life habits provides more information about undergraduate educators to enable higher education institutions to redirect their activities according to the characteristics of their teaching staff. In addition to the theoretical models of quality of life, the concept and constructs of personality, emotions and the presence of a negative dimension influence quality of life in such a way that studying it has become a challenge today, incorporating social, cross-cultural aspects, conceptual, methodological, psychometric and statistical studies. However, it is necessary to broaden the discussion on teachers' quality of life (CONCEIÇÂO *et al.,* 2012).

There is a need to work towards improving teachers' working conditions in order to reduce the psychic suffering to which they are exposed, improve the degree of satisfaction in their family, love, social and environmental lives and, consequently, in their professional activity, which contributes to a better quality of life (OLIVEIRA *et al.*, 2012).

Thus, considering that the university space may or may not cause experiences that contribute to the quality of life of these professionals, it is important to carry out this research so that it can support, as a source of information, the development of support and coping strategies for health teachers and the implementation of formalized spaces geared to their real realities to offer opportunities to resolve difficult situations in their daily lives and promote health and quality of life. This study could also be a stimulus for other studies to assess the quality of life of health teachers in other settings.

In this context, the aim of this study was to assess the quality of life of teachers in undergraduate health courses at a public university.

CHAPTER 3

METHODOLOGY

3.1 THEORETICAL-METHODOLOGICAL FOUNDATION

This was a descriptive, quantitative study with a cross-sectional and analytical design.

According to Gil (2010) scientific research is a rational and systematic procedure that aims to provide answers to the problems that are proposed, in which it is required when there is not enough information to answer a particular problem. For Barros and Lehfeld (2009), it is the product of an investigation, the aim of which is to solve problems and resolve doubts through the use of scientific procedures.

In the health field, according to Polit, Beck and Hungler (2011), research is aimed at developing knowledge on issues of importance to professionals and includes practice, teaching and administration. It allows us to generate new knowledge, guide professional practice, improve care and the quality of life of health service users, establish professional identity and also describe characteristics of particular situations that have not been explored much.

This study is characterized as exploratory because, according to Gil (2010), exploratory research aims to provide greater familiarity with the problem in order to make it more explicit. The first stage of all scientific research does not aim to immediately solve a problem, but only to understand and characterize it.

It is also a descriptive study because it is in line with Gil (2010), who refers to this type of research as the description of the characteristics of a given population or phenomenon, or the establishment of relationships between variables, which may be associated, and the facts are observed, recorded, analyzed, classified and interpreted, without the researcher interfering in them, i.e. the phenomena are studied, but not manipulated by the researcher.

The quantitative approach, used in this research, is interested in the facts detected and observable, ensuring the objectivity and credibility of these findings. It refers to closed scientific knowledge, generally unchanged, in which it seeks hypothetical-deductive explanation to test objective theories, examining the relationship between variables. These variables can typically be measured by instruments, so that the data obtained can be analyzed by statistical procedures (COSTA, M.; COSTA, B., 2012; CRESWELL, 2010).

The research design refers to the planning of the investigation in its broadest sense, involving both its layout and the forecast for analyzing and interpreting the data. The most important element in identifying a design is the procedure adopted for data collection. To this end, this study uses *surveys*, which are characterized by direct questioning of individuals whose opinions and behaviour we wish to know. Information is requested from a significant group of people about the problem studied and then, through quantitative analysis, the corresponding conclusions are drawn from the data collected, allowing direct knowledge of reality (GIL, 2010).

3.2 CHARACTERIZATION OF THE RESEARCH SITE

This research was carried out at the Center for Biological and Health Sciences on the campus of a public university, with teachers from the undergraduate courses in Biological Sciences (BA), Biological Sciences (BSc), Physical Education (BSc), Physical Education (BSc), Medicine and Dentistry.

This university was created in 1962 by State Law No. 2.615/1962, and in 1963 it became the first higher education institution in the north of Minas Gerais. It was called the Faculty of Philosophy, Sciences and Letters (FAFIL). From 1963 to 1990, the Faculties of Law (FADIR), Economics (FADEC), Medicine (FAMED) and Arts (FACEART) were created. In order to comply with the provisions of the State Constitution, State Decree no. 30.971, of 09/03/90 "instituted the State University of Montes Claros", and its first Statute was approved by State Decree no. 31.840, of 24/09/1990 (UNIMONTES, 2008).

State Law No. 11.517, of 13/07/94, reorganized UNIMONTES from an administrative-functional point of view. The Faculties were abolished and the Teaching Centres were created: the Human Sciences Centre (CCH), the Biological and Health Sciences Centre, the Applied Social Sciences Centre (CCSA), the Exact and Technological

Sciences Centre and the Secondary and Fundamental Education Centre (CEMF). The Center for Biological and Health Sciences is home to the Departments of Biological Sciences, Physical Education, Nursing, Medicine and Dentistry (UNIMONTES, 1999).

The degree course in Biological Sciences is offered in two forms: Bachelor's and Bachelor's degrees. The first was established in 1996 by Resolution 004/96 of the University Council, and was recognized by Decree No. 41743/01 of the Minas Gerais State Education Council (CEEMG). The basic characteristic of this course is the training of professionals capable of applying their knowledge together with available technologies to the rational sustainable use of natural resources, associated with the maintenance and balance of ecosystems and sanitation, with the aim of preserving life in all its forms and manifestations. The course offers two options: a Bachelor's Degree in Biotechnology, with an emphasis on biotechnology and/or a Bachelor's Degree in Conservation Biology, with an emphasis on the environment. It takes four years to complete, with classes held in the daytime (morning and afternoon), enrollment is on a semester basis, 40 places are offered per year and it has 58 teaching staff. Also created in 1996, by Resolution 004/96 of the University Council, the Degree Course in Biological Sciences aims to train qualified professionals to work as teachers in primary and secondary schools, and as researchers who are able to visualize possibilities for action associated with the needs of the region, and to take on responsibilities in the field of teaching and research. This course has a minimum duration of eight terms and a maximum of 14, classes are held in the evening, the enrollment regime is also semester-based, 35 semester places are available and it is made up of 58 teachers.

The degree course in Physical Education is offered in Bachelor's and Licentiate's degrees. The Bachelor's Degree in Physical Education was created in 1994 by means of Resolution No. 11 - CEPEX/94 of 18/08/94, and was recognized by Decree No. 41.411 of 06/12/2000. The course lasts four years, with daytime classes and semester enrollment. 21 places are on offer and it has 54 teaching staff. Graduates in Physical Education should be able to plan, implement and lead physical activities aimed at developing physical fitness related to the motor skills of children, adolescents, adults and the elderly, related to well-being and health maintenance. In order to train professionals with technical-functional and didactic-pedagogical knowledge who are able to intervene competently, critically and creatively in the school context, the Degree Course in Physical Education/Licenciatura was created by means of Resolution No. 11 - CEPEX/94 of 18/08/94 and recognized by Decree 41.411 of 06/12/2000. This course has a semester enrollment system, offers 53 places for the evening and 21 places for the day, and is made up of 53 teachers.

Authorization for the creation of the Bachelor's Degree in Medicine was granted in 1974 by Federal Decree 74.844 of November 6, 1974. The primary characteristic of the course is to train professionals who are able to face the challenges of the new millennium, especially with regard to finding solutions to the health problems that afflict humanity, essentially contributing with broad knowledge in preventive, care and curative medicine, with an emphasis on the areas of clinical medicine, clinical surgery, pediatrics, gynecology and obstetrics and social medicine. The course lasts six years, with full time teaching, offers 28 places per semester and is made up of 177 teachers.

The Dentistry Degree Course was established in 1994 by means of Resolution No. 11 - CEPEX/94, of 18/08/94, Opinion CEPEX 024/94 and Resolution No. 10 - University Council/94, of 01/09/94. Its aim is to provide the job market with professionals who have solid knowledge to exercise their profession ethically and competently, valuing the national reality and promoting health; and with the ability to act as a dental surgeon and general practitioner, in individual and collective preventive aspects, curing and repairing oral and dental diseases and public health. The course has 10 periods with full-time classes, semester enrollment, offers 24 places and is made up of 67 teachers.

In this context, the study was carried out with teachers from undergraduate courses in Biological Sciences (Bachelor's Degree), Biological Sciences (Bachelor's Degree), Physical Education (Bachelor's Degree), Physical Education (Bachelor's Degree), Medicine and Dentistry at the Center for Biological and Health Sciences on the main campus of a public university, who freely agreed to sign the Informed Consent Form (ANNEX A) regarding their participation; making this the ideal place to carry out this research.

3.3 POPULATION AND SAMPLE

The target population of the study was teachers from the following courses: Biological Sciences - Bachelor's Degree, Biological Sciences - Degree, Physical Education - Bachelor's Degree, Physical Education - Degree, Nursing, Medicine and Dentistry, located on the campus of a public university. The number of teachers at the Center for Biological and Health Sciences is shown in TAB.1.

Table 1. Number of professors in undergraduate health courses at a public university in Minas Gerais, 2012.

Degree Course	**No. of Periods**	**No. of teachers**
Biological Sciences: Bachelor's Degree	8	58
Physical Education: BA and BSc	8	53
Medicine / Bachelor	12	177
Dentistry / Bachelor	10	67
Total	-	**355**

Source: Human Resources Development Department - 2012.

As a criterion for inclusion, the teachers had to be involved in teaching activities in the undergraduate courses. We excluded those who were on leave for the following reasons: studying for a post-graduate *degree* or doctorate, maternity leave, statutory leave, leave for health treatment, retirement, premium leave and leave to attend to private interests.

There were 43 Biological Sciences, 43 Physical Education, 65 Nursing, 165 Medicine and 63 Dentistry teachers in the study, totaling 379. Stratified probability sampling was used to define the sample, and participants were selected at random. The calculations used in this sample were based on a conservative prevalence of 50% for positive quality of life averages, a population of 379 teachers, a margin of error of 3.5% and a 95% confidence level. The number identified was increased by 15% for possible losses. Thus, the minimum number of teachers for the study defined by the sample calculation was 295 individuals, who were identified by random drawing from each stratum, i.e. each course.

3.4 INSTRUMENT AND DATA COLLECTION

The instrument used for data collection was the generic questionnaire on quality of life from the World Health Organization (WHO), called the *World Health Organization's Abbreviated Quality of Life Assessment Tool* (WHOQOL-Bref), which consists of the abbreviated version of the WHOQOL-100 (ANNEX B), developed by the WHO Quality of Life Group, according to Fleck *et al.* (2000). The WHOQOL-100 resulted from a multi-center collaborative project with the aim of building an instrument that would assess quality of life from an international perspective (FLECK *et al.*, 1999). The abbreviated version was created in response to the need for instruments that required less time to complete and that maintained the quality of the WHOQOL-100's psychometric characteristics (WHOQOL GROUP, 2000). The instrument, in its abbreviated version, was validated by Professor Marcelo Fleck, coordinator of the WHOQOL Group, by means of an extensive study carried out in the state of Rio Grande do Sul in 1998. The WHOQOL-bref was created to assess quality of life from an international perspective, translated into 50 languages and used in 51 countries (CONCEIÇÂO *et al.,* 2012).

The Portuguese version of the WHOQOL-bref was developed at the WHOQOL Center for Brazil and contains 26 questions: two general questions, which are not included in the calculation of the domain scores, one referring to LIFE and the other to HEALTH. The remaining 24 questions relate to the four domains and their respective facets, as follows: Domain I - *physical*, focusing on the following facets: pain and discomfort, energy and fatigue, sleep and rest, activities of daily living, dependence on medication or treatment, ability to work; Domain II - *psychological*, whose facets are: positive feelings, thinking, learning, memory and concentration, self-esteem, body image and appearance, negative feelings, spirituality, religiosity and personal beliefs; Domain III - *social relations*, which includes the following facets: personal relationships, social support, sexual activity; Domain IV - *environment*, covering the facets: physical safety and protection, home environment, financial resources, health and social care, availability and quality, opportunities to acquire new information and skills, participation in, and opportunities for recreation/leisure, physical environment - pollution, noise, traffic, climate, transportation. This instrument considers the last fifteen days experienced by the respondents. The answers to the questions are given on a scale with a single interval from 0 (zero) to 5 (five), according to the WHOQOL methodology (FLECK *et al*., 2000; ALVES *et al.,* 2010.).

The answers to each question that makes up the domain result in final scores ranging from 4 to 20, which can be transformed into 0 to 100, measured in a positive direction. Higher scores indicate a better assessment of quality of life (FLECK *et al*., 2000).

The WHOQOL-bref was chosen for this study because it has been developed and validated, showing satisfactory psychometric characteristics (FLECK *et al*., 2000), which are important when choosing an instrument to assess quality of life (PASCHOAL, 2001). The WHOQOL-bref has been used in different countries and with different groups of people, demonstrating its many possibilities for use in an international and cross-cultural perspective (KLUTHCOVSKY, A.; KLUTHCOVSKY, F., 2009).

The Portuguese version - including the questionnaires - is available in Brazil at the Quality of Life Study Group of the Department of Psychiatry at the Federal University of Rio Grande do Sul and at the Hospital das Clinicas do Paranâ. The results of the process of validating the Portuguese version of the WHOQOL-Bref were carried out along the same lines as the validation process for the WHOQOL-100 in Brazil and in other research centers and showed good psychometric performance with satisfactory characteristics of internal consistency, discriminant validity, criterion validity, concurrent validity and test-retest reliability (FLECK *et al*., 1999; FLECK *et al*., 2000).

In a descriptive-exploratory study, in which the LILACS and MEDLINE databases were searched in order to carry out a literature review on studies that used the WHOQOL-bref as an instrument for collecting data in quality of life assessments, Kluthcovsky, A. and Kluthcovsky, F. (2009) selected 169 abstracts of articles published on the subject up to December 31, 2006, constituting the base material for the analysis. The first study was published in 1998 and found a progressive increase in the number of studies using the WHOQOL-bref over the years, especially in 2005 and 2006 (62.1% of the total). The countries that published the most studies of this type were Brazil (14.2%), followed by Taiwan (13%) and Germany (8.2%). Several journals have published on the subject, with Quality of Life Research predominating, with 31 articles (18.3%). Of the 107 journals, 29.8% were related to the fields of psychiatry, psychology and mental health. As for the aims of the studies, the majority referred to validating or evaluating the psychometric properties of the WHOQOL-bref, followed by evaluating quality of life in a group of subjects and their respective subgroups and evaluating quality of life in a group of subjects compared to a control group.

The information obtained through questionnaires makes it possible to observe the characteristics of an individual or a group, benefiting the analysis to be carried out by the researcher, as well as allowing the measurement of individual or group variables. Such questionnaires can include single and multiple questions.

The authors concluded that the WHOQOL-bref can be used in clinical practice as a way of improving the doctor-patient relationship, as a tool for evaluating and comparing responses to different treatments, in evaluations of health services , in research and in evaluating health policies. It is a short, quick-to-apply instrument that can be used both in populations with some kind of disease and in healthy populations. This points to the possibility of carrying out several other future studies on different populations that have already been studied or not, especially in Brazil, which has stood out among other countries in terms of the use of the WHOQOL-bref. These studies can generate new knowledge, raise questions and contribute to making decisions that will improve people's quality of life.

In this study, additional information was also collected on the university's undergraduate health teachers regarding sociodemographic aspects, in order to describe their profile and establish associations with quality of life when analyzing the data (APPENDIX A). The variables relating to socio-demographic aspects contained in this second questionnaire were analyzed using absolute and relative frequencies and descriptive statistical measures. After checking the normality of these variables, Student's *t-test* was used to compare means and Fisher's exact test to compare proportions. The level of statistical significance adopted was 5%.

The two instruments were applied on the premises of the Center for Biological and

Health Sciences, in the classroom or in another environment agreed in advance with the teachers and at a pre-established time so as not to interfere with their teaching activities. Before collecting the data, a pilot study was carried out to test the instruments to be used. During the pilot study, the researcher took notes of the interviewees' reactions, degree of difficulty in understanding and embarrassment about the questions.

questions. It also makes it possible to check for unnecessary, superfluous and inappropriate questions and has the main function of testing the data instrument (MEDEIROS, 2009; GIL, 2010). A pilot study was therefore carried out with three professors from different areas of health, from another Higher Education Institution, one from the 1st period, one from the 5th and one from the 10th, in order to ascertain the time taken to answer the questionnaires, the degree of understanding and the difficulties encountered by the participants related to the interpretation of some questions, the definition of unfamiliar words and to check whether the instrument meets the objectives proposed by the study. In view of the difficulties pointed out, the researchers made the necessary changes in order to improve the consistency of the answers.

The instrument was applied by the researchers themselves, who provided additional explanations to the questionnaires at the time of data collection. Appointments were made in advance with the coordinators of the Biological Sciences Bachelor's Degree, Biological Sciences Bachelor's Degree, Physical Education Bachelor's Degree, Physical Education Bachelor's Degree, Medicine and Dentistry courses. The objectives of the research were explained and clarification was given regarding the confidentiality of individual data.

Questionnaires are a method of collecting data in the field, of interacting with interviewees through an ordered series of questions and situations that you want to investigate (VERGARA, 2009). Like any other data collection method, the questionnaire has numerous possibilities and also limitations. One of the possibilities of the questionnaire is that it can cover more information and obtain it in a shorter space of time than interviews and observations. When they are closed, as in this research, it allows results to be compared with each other, considering that the questions and answers are standardized. It also allows for anonymity and helps to reduce costs, since all participants can take part in the collection at once, in a previously organized location (VERGARA, 2009; BARROS, LEHFELD, 2009; GIL, 2010).

To this end, in this investigation, care was taken to ensure that the answers were reliable, relevant and contributed to the ongoing process of generating knowledge, as recommended by Vergara (2009). Data collection took place after approval of this research project by the Research Ethics Committee of the university campus of a public university and authorization from the Director of the Centre for Biological and Health Sciences, the Heads of Departments and the Coordinators of the Bachelor's Degree Courses in Biological Sciences, Biological Sciences Bachelor's Degree, Physics Education Bachelor's Degree, Physics Education Bachelor's Degree, Medicine and Dentistry to carry out this research and through the Institution's Term of Agreement for Participation in Research (ANNEX C), which was signed by the Director of the Center for Biological and Health Sciences.

3.5 DATA ORGANIZATION AND ANALYSIS

After collection, the data was organized in a database using the *Statistical Package for the Social Science* (SPSS) Windows 19.0® version.

In this study, we considered the distribution of quality of life scores according to the domains analyzed: poor quality of life (21-40); neither poor nor good (41-60); good (61-80) and very good, when the scores ranged from 8-1100.

The questions (1) How do you rate your quality of life? (very bad; bad; neither bad nor good; good; very good) and (2) How satisfied are you with your health? (very dissatisfied; dissatisfied; neither satisfied nor dissatisfied; satisfied; very satisfied) were analyzed separately because they are not included in the equations for the Whoqol syntax.

The covariates were grouped into sociodemographic and academic characteristics. The covariates included gender, age (dichotomized using the mean as the cut-off point), marital status (categorized as married and stable union and without a partner, including single and widowed), self-declared color (categorized as brown and other, including white, black and indigenous). In addition to place of birth and residence, who they live with (categorized as living with their own family and another situation - living with friends or alone), family income which was categorized by the average, other employment (yes and no), length of time teaching, categorized based on the average. We also investigated whether they read books, except for academics, whether they have a computer with internet access at home, and whether they use the internet as their main source of information, both categorized as yes or no. It was also assessed whether the teacher, apart from academic activities, is more involved in cultural activities, including going to the theater, cinema, parks and leisure time with friends, or social and family activities - usually staying at home, watching TV and attending family events.

After collection, the data was organized and analyzed using the *Statistical Package for Social Sciences* (SPSS) 18.0. Descriptive statistics were used to analyze the data, using absolute and relative frequencies and calculating means and standard deviations. In order to investigate associations between sociodemographic and academic variables and the quality of life domains, the normality of the data was checked using the *Klomogorov-Smirnov* test. Bivariate analysis was then carried out, using the *Student's* t-test for independent samples and *Bonferroni*'s *ANOVA/post hoc* variables with three or more categories to compare the mean quality of life scores in each domain. The purpose of these tests was to compare the mean scores in each domain in relation to the covariates. A significance level of 5% ($p \leq 0.05$) was used in all analyses.

3.6 ETHICAL ASPECTS

The interest in ethics applied to life is growing as we reflect on the conflicts between biotechnology and life. Scientific research triggers a demanding biological moral reflection and, consequently, a new system in which dialog and discussion play an indispensable role in the elaboration, execution and development of research on living beings (MARCOS, 1999).

In this context, the ethical aspects of this research were considered in accordance with Resolution 466/2012 of the National Research Ethics Committee of the Ministry of Health, which stipulates ethical standards for research involving human beings. To this end, a research project was drawn up and approved by the Research Ethics Committee. Authorization was sought from the Director of the Center for Biological and Health Sciences, the Heads of Departments and the Coordinators of the Biological Sciences Bachelor's Degree, Biological Sciences Bachelor's Degree, Physical Education Bachelor's Degree, Physical Education Degree, Nursing, Medicine and Dentistry as to whether this research would be carried out, by means of the Institution's Term of Agreement for Participation in Research (ANNEX C), which was signed by the Director of the Center for Biological and Health Sciences.

In accordance with the norms of Resolution 466/2012, this study was approved by the Research Ethics Committee, through Consubstantiated Opinion 173.395/2012, Certificate of Submission for Ethical Appraisal (CAAE) 10944812.3.0000.5146. All participants signed an informed consent form.

Before the data collection instrument was distributed for completion, the subjects of the study signed the Informed Consent Form (ANNEX A), which was also signed by the study coordinator and a witness. The content of the form was previously explained and discussed with the participants, as was the purpose and reason for the research, the justification for choosing the participants and the guarantee of anonymity and confidentiality of the data collected.

The data collection instruments were applied by the researchers themselves, who gave additional explanations at the time of data collection in the room and/or at another location, at a time previously scheduled with the Coordinators of the Biological Sciences Bachelor's Degree, Biological Sciences Bachelor's Degree, Physical Education Bachelor's Degree, Physical Education Bachelor's Degree, Medicine and Dentistry Courses.

CHAPTER 4

RESULTS

Of the total of 295 teachers defined by the sample calculation, 221 answered the questionnaires, giving a response rate of 75%. Thus, 34 (15.4%) biology teachers, 35 (15.8%) physical education teachers, 50 (22.6%) dentistry teachers, 48 (21.7%) medical teachers and 54 (24.4%) nursing teachers took part in the study.

4.1 sociodemographic characteristics

The sociodemographic characteristics of the teachers of undergraduate health courses were as follows: the majority were female in biology (67.6%), dentistry (56.0%), medicine (56.3%) and nursing (77.8%). However, in the physical education course, the majority of teachers were male (51.4%). The age group up to 43 years was predominant among the teachers of all the courses in question - biology 58.8%, physical education 60.0%, dentistry 52.0%, medicine 51.0% and nursing 72.2%.

As for marital status, the majority of teachers from all courses were married - biology 67.6%, physical education 74.3%, dentistry 82.0%, medicine 70.8%, nursing 64.8%. In addition, the teachers declared themselves to be white (biology 55.9%, physical education 57.1%, dentistry 62.0%, medicine 58.3%, nursing 51.0%); live in the city of Montes Claros (biology 70.6%, physical education 100.0%, dentistry 96.0%, medicine 100.0%, nursing 98.1%) and live with their families (biology 70.6%, physical education 85.7%, dentistry 94.0%, medicine 85.4%, nursing 85.2%).

With regard to having another employment relationship, teachers in physical education (51.4%), dentistry (60.0%), medicine (85.4%) and nursing (75.9%) said they had more than one. However, among the biology teachers, 32.4% had another job. With regard to the length of time they have been teaching, the majority have been teaching for up to 12 years - biology 58.8%, physical education 62.9%, dentistry 62.0%, nursing 72.2%. However, in the medicine course, it was observed that the majority had 13 years or more of teaching experience (60.4%).

In addition, the majority have a gross monthly income of up to 11 minimum wages -

biology 64.7%, physical education 68.6%, dentistry 62.0% and nursing 66.7%. On the other hand, in the medicine course, the majority of teachers had a gross income of more than 12 minimum wages (64.6%).

With regard to university education, the majority have a master's degree - biology 79.4%, physical education 54.3%, dentistry 70.0%, medicine 54.2% and nursing 59.3%; they read more than two books a year, excluding academic bibliography - biology 70.6%, physical education 54.3%, dentistry 56.0%, medicine 50.2% and nursing 63.0%.

Most of the teachers were non-smokers - biology 79.4%, physical education 88.6%, dentistry 92.0%, medicine 97.9% and nursing 100.0%; they have other sources of information besides the internet - biology 61.8%, physical education 71.4%, dentistry 82.0%, medicine 68.8% and nursing 59.3%.

With regard to leisure activities, the majority prefer cultural activities - physical education 74.3%, dentistry 62.0%, medicine 54.2% and nursing 63.0%; except for biology teachers, who prefer social activities (55.9%) (TABLE 2).

Table 2. Socio-demographic profile of teachers, Montes Claros-MG, 2014 (n=221).

Variable	N (221)	%
Sex		
Male	84	38
Female	137	62
Age		
Up to 43 years old	130	58,8
44 or more	91	41,2
Marital status		
With a partner	159	71,9
Without a partner	62	28,1
Race		
White	125	56,6
Brown and others	96	43,4
Where you live		
In Montes Claros	217	98,2
Other	4	1,8
Who you live with		
With his own family	188	85,1
Another situation	33	14,9
Other employment No	80	36,2
Yes	141	63,8
Length of time teaching		
Up to 12 years old	134	60,6
Over 12 years old	87	39,4

Gross Monthly Income		
Up to 11 salaries	130	58,8
Above 11 salaries	91	41,2
Maximum level of university education		
With a master's degree	130	58,8
No master's degree	82	37,1
Books other than academic books		
Up to 2 books	92	41,6
More than 2 books	179	58,4
Smoker		
No	205	92,8
Yes	16	7,2
Source of information Internet	81	36,7
Other sources	140	63,3
Leisure		
Social activities	89	40,3
Cultural activities	132	59,7

4.2 QUALITY OF LIFE FOR TEACHERS

With regard to general quality of life, the majority of teachers (75.1%) rated their health as good. With regard to how satisfied teachers are with their own health, the majority (69.7%) said they were satisfied with their health.

The results obtained from the WHOQOL responses were expressed as means and standard deviations of the transformed scores (percentages), calculated in advance for each of the domains. The greatest variation in standard deviation occurred in the "social relations" domain and the least in the "physical" domain, which was the most affected, as it had the lowest mean values (57.9; SD±9.6); while "social relations" with the highest value (73.7; SD±17.2) was the most positive aspect of teachers' quality of life. In relation to the course of study, the highest mean scores were found among dentistry teachers in the physical (60.3; SD+10.9) and environmental (73.9; SD+15.7) domains. Higher scores were identified in the psychological (69.7; SD+ 9.3) and social relations (78.8; SD+ 5.0) domains in the physical education course (TABLE 3).

Table 3 Mean and standard deviation scores for the quality of life domains (WHOQOL/breve) of teachers at a public university in Minas Gerais, 2014 (n=221).

Domains	**Biology**	**Physical Education**	**Dentistry**	**Medicine**	**Nursing**	**Overall Average**
Physical	55,1 + 8,0	58,5 + 9,0	60,3 + 10,9	60,0 + 9,6	57,8 + 8,8	57,9 + 9,6
Psychological	64,8 + 1,3	69,7 + 9,3	66,6 + 11,7	65,6 + 0,6	66,5 + 11,5	66,6 + 1,1
Social relations	71,3 + 2,8	78,8 + 5,0	78,0 + 16,9	68,4 + 8,1	72,5 + 18,9	73,7 +17,2
Environment	65,0 + 0,9	73,0+ 4,7	73,9 + 15,7	68,3 +14,5	71,0 + 11,4	70,4 +13,9

4.3 ASSOCIATIONS OF QUALITY OF LIFE SCORES WITH TEACHERS' SOCIODEMOGRAPHIC AND ACADEMIC CHARACTERISTICS

Table 4 shows the association between quality of life scores and the teachers' sociodemographic characteristics. There was a statistically significant association (p=0.037) between the physical domain and age, with higher scores, 59.5 (SD±9.1) for those aged 44 or over, i.e. in this domain, older people have a better quality of life than younger people.

With regard to marital status, there were significant associations in the psychological (p=0.009), social relations (p=0.041) and environmental (p=0.034) domains, with higher mean scores for those with a partner, i.e. those with a better quality of life. The fact of living with one's family determined a higher average score, 74.6 (SD±14.2), for the social relations domain (p=0.04). In relation to leisure, there was a statistically significant association in the social relations (p=0.039) and environment (p=0.045) domains, with higher scores, respectively 76.6 (SD±16.2) and 72.7 (SD±13.4), for those who spend more time on social activities, indicating a better quality of life for these individuals compared to those who spend more time on cultural activities. Higher income was associated with higher quality of life scores, 72.9 (SD±13.2) in the environment domain (p=0.029).

Table 4

Average scores in the quality of life domains according to the sociodemographic characteristics of teachers at a public university. Montes Claros (MG), Brazil. 2014 (n = 221).

Average quality of life scores

Variables	n (%)	Physical	Psychological	Social Relations	Environment
Sex					
Female	128 (57,9)	57,7	65,9	72,4	70,6
Male	93 (42,1)	58,2	67,7	75,7	70,2
p - value (t-test)		0,74	0,23	0,17	0,81
Age					
Up to 43 years old	130 (58,8)	56,8	65,8	74,3	69,5
44 or more	91 (41,2)	59,5	67,9	72,7	71,9
p - value (t-test)		**0,03**	0,16	0,48	0,21
Marital status					
With a partner	159 (71,9)	58,5	67,9	75,1	71,7
Without a partner	62 (28,1)	56,3	63,5	69,8	63,3
p - value (t-test)		0,13	**0,00**	**0,04**	**0,03**
Self-declared color	125 (56,6)	58,2	66,4	74,7	71

White					
Brown and others	96 (43,4)	57,5	67	72,4	69,7
p - value (t-test)		0, 58	0,68	0,33	0,48
Where you live					
In Montes Claros	217 (98,2)	57,9	66,6	73,7	70,5
Other	4 (1,8)	59,4	64,6	72,9	67,9
p - value (t-test)		0,76	0,71	0,92	0,71
Who you live with					
With family	188 (85,1)	58	67,1	74,6	70,9
Another situation	33 (14,9)	57,6	63,8	68,2	67,6
p - value (t-test)		0,82	0,10	**0,04**	0,20
Leisure					
Social activities	89 (40,3)	58,14	68,1	76,6	72,7
Cultural activities	132 (59,7)	57,8	65,6	71,7	68,9
p - value (t-test)		0,77	0,10	**0,03**	**0,04**
Gross Monthly Income					
Above 11 salaries	130 (58,8)	58,2	67,5	73,8	72,9
Up to 11 salaries	91 (41,2)	57,7	66,0	73,6	68,7
p - value (t-test)		0,72	0,33	0,92	**0,02**

As shown in Table 5, in relation to the type of course in which the teacher works, there were statistically significant differences in the social relations and environment domains. Higher mean quality of life scores were observed for physical education teachers, 78.8 (SD±5.0), and lower for medicine teachers, 68.4 (SD±8.1), in the social relations domain (p=0.010). In the environment domain (p=0.030), physical education teachers had higher scores, 73.9 (SD±4.7), while biology teachers had lower scores, 65.0 (SD±0.9). With regard to length of teaching experience, there was a statistically significant association in the physical, psychological and environmental domains, with higher scores for teachers with up to 12 years of teaching experience. Thus, teachers with less time in the teaching profession have a higher quality of life.

There was also a statistically significant association between the number of books read each year, with the exception of academic books, and the physical (p=0.002) and psychological (p=0.013) domains, with higher scores, 59.6 (SD±9.3) for physical and 68.2 (SD±11.1) for psychological, for those who read up to two books a year.

As for the other characteristics - gender, self-declared color, place of residence, other employment, maximum level of university education, smoker, source of information - no significant associations were found.

Table 5

Average scores in the quality of life domains according to the academic characteristics of teachers at a public university. Montes Claros (MG), Brazil. 2014 (n = 221)

Average quality of life scores					
Variables	**n (%)**	**Physical**	**Psychological**	**Social Relations**	**Environment**
Course					
Biology	34 (15,4)	55,1	64,8	71,3	65,0
Physical Education	35 (15,8)	58,7	69,7	78,8	73,9
Dentistry	50 (22,6)	60,3	66,6	78,0	73,0
Medicine	48 (21,7)	56,9	65,6	68,4	68,3
Nursing	54 (24,4)	57,8	66,5	72,5	71,0
p - value (Anova)		0,15	0,39	**0,01**	**0,03**
Other employment					
No	80 (36,2)	58,01	67,5	76,35	71,2
Yes	141 (63,8)	57,9	66,1	72,2	70,0
p - value (t-test)		0,90	0,35	0,08	0,53
Length of time teaching					
Up to 12 years old	134 (60,6)	59,6	68,7	75,1	72,8
Over 12 years old	87 (39,4)	56,8	65,3	72,8	68,9
p - value (t-test)		**0,03**	**0,02**	0,32	**0,04**
Maximum level of university education					
With a *post-graduate* degree	130 (58,8)	57,8	66,6	74,2	12,7
No postgraduate *degree*	82 (37,1)	58,1	66,7	72,8	70,7
p - value (t-test)		0,80	0,96	0,54	0,84
Books, except academic ones					
Up to 2 books	92 (41,6)	59,6	68,2	74,6	71,6
More than 2 books	179 (58,4)	55,6	64,4	72,4	68,9
p - value (t-test)		**0,00**	**0,01**	0,34	0,15

CHAPTER 5

DISCUSSION

The sociodemographic profile of the teachers taking part in this study was similar to that found in other studies on this subject (DAVILA; CASAGRANDE; PEREIRA, 2010; FERNANDES; ROCHA; FAGUNDES, 2011; DAMASIO; MELO; SILVA, 2013).

With regard to quality of life, this study showed a good quality of life in the psychological, social relations and environmental domains. However, the physical domain was found to be fair. A similar study carried out in a Higher Education Institution in the south of Brazil, using the WHOQOL-Breve, with the aim of assessing the perception of quality of life and health and risk factors of 293 teachers, also found that there was a higher score for the psychological, social relations and environment domains, with values similar to those found in the present study (FILHO; NETTO-OLIVEIRA; OLIVEIRA, 2012).

Research carried out among 517 teachers from public and private institutions in the city of Campina Grande (Paraiba), to assess the sense of life, psychological well-being and quality of life indices in a sample of educators, showed different results to those found in this study, since the psychological and social domains showed regular quality of life. This shows the need to look closely at the health of teachers in this scenario (DAMASIO; MELO; SILVA, 2013). On the other hand, this study obtained good results for the psychological, social relations and environmental domains.

A study similar to this one, carried out with 203 teachers in Rio Grande do Sul, with the aim of investigating the quality of life of teachers at community higher education institutions, identified an average of 71.3 in the social relations domain, similar to that found in this investigation, i.e. quality of life, as in this study, was also good among teachers in Rio Grande do Sul (KOETZ; REMPEL; PÉRICO, 2013).

There is a study carried out at the University of Vale do Itajai (UNIVALI), in Santa Catarina, which, when assessing the quality of life of teachers, found that the environment domain obtained the second lowest score, different from the data found in this research (COGO *et al.,* 2011).

When the domains were associated with sociodemographic variables, in this study, age had a higher average score in the physical domain for teachers aged over 44. Similar data was found among 203 teachers from universities in Rio Grande do Sul, in which teachers aged over 40 had a better quality of life (KOETZ; REMPEL; PÉRICO, 2013). However, it is worth noting that the physical domain includes aspects such as pain and discomfort, sleep and rest, activities of daily living and work capacity. These aspects tend to be compromised by advancing age, negatively affecting quality of life, as revealed in a study carried out in another public institution also in southern Brazil, where more negative perceptions of health increased with age (FILHO; NETTO-OLIVEIRA; OLIVEIRA, 2012).

In this study, the marital status variable obtained significant data in the psychological, social relations and environmental domains, with higher scores for teachers who had a partner. A similar study carried out in the state of Rio Grande do Sul, with the aim of analyzing the individual and socio-environmental parameters of the perceived quality of life in a career, with 380 educators, showed that married teachers had a good quality of life18. A study carried out in Natal (RN) also showed similar data to this study, in which married teachers have a better quality of life (FERNANDES; ROCHA; FAGUNDES, 2011).

It has been observed that married teachers, who supposedly have an established family routine, can adopt healthier behaviors compared to their colleagues in the same profession who don't have a partner. Despite this, the latter don't have to worry too much about satisfying the wishes, expectations and desires of a formal partner and/or their dependent(s) (SALLES *et al.*, 2012). However, this reality may be different for men and women, but this study found no significant difference between the sexes.

In another study, which aimed to analyze the perception of quality of life and health and the incidence of modifiable risk factors in teachers at a public higher education institution in southern Brazil, it was observed that university teachers with a good economic level had a better quality of life in the environmental domain (FILHO; NETTO-OLIVEIRA; OLIVEIRA, 2012). In this study, gross monthly income above 11 minimum wages favored a higher score in the environment domain, which confirms the similarities between the findings. From this perspective, salary and professional appreciation are factors that can provide better living conditions and a better quality of life (DAVILA; CASAGRANDE; PEREIRA, 2010). When investigating the value placed on the teaching profession in the academic sphere, both in the perception of the social imaginary and in job, career and salary plans, it can be seen that teachers in public higher education are in a good position. For this reason, the result was positive for most of the participants in this survey, in terms of the remuneration and stability achieved through their current employment relationship (LAGO; CUNHA; BORGES, 2015).

The association between the domains and the academic variables in this study showed that educators who had been teaching for less than 12 years achieved higher scores in the physical, psychological and environmental domains. In a similar study assessing the quality of life of 73 students using the WHOQOL-Breve in Maceió (AL), it was found that a shorter teaching career was associated with higher quality of life scores in the physical domain, similar to the findings of the present study (MORAIS; AZEVEDO; CHIARI, 2012). The conjecture for these findings is more favorable for professionals with shorter careers, who may enjoy better health conditions and greater willingness to perform work activities. On the other hand, it is pertinent to reflect that teachers who have been working for longer and are older generally feel more secure, emotionally and professionally stable, cope better with diversity, have a better understanding of the position of colleagues, academics and managers, and their expectations are different (KOETZ; REMPEL; PÉRICO, 2013). Despite the fact that this context contributes positively to their quality of life, in this study, older teachers had lower scores in the aforementioned quality of life domains.

It was also found that those who live with their families have a good quality of life. However, in an investigation carried out with 349 teachers in Florianópolis (SC), also using the WHOQOL-Breve, with the aim of investigating teachers' perception of quality of life, a lower quality of life score was found for people who live with their family (PEREIRA; TEIXEIRA; LOPES, 2013). Even considering that the dual routine of teachers can lead to family and health problems, it is understood that the family is of great importance for the development of its members. Everyone needs to be involved so that they can perform their duties satisfactorily (SILVA; ARPINI, 2013).

The professional practice of teaching is marked by factors and feelings that compromise quality of life in general. Assessing quality of life is a first step towards reflecting on these aspects and sharing the situations that influence it positively or negatively. As soon as teachers are made aware of situations that affect their quality of life, they can start looking for better living and working conditions (COGO *et al.*, 2011).

The physical education teachers obtained higher scores in the social relations and environment domains, while the medicine and biology teachers obtained lower scores. This finding is in line with research into the experience of teaching in health courses at a federal university in the northern region of Brazil. Although professional practice has been identified as a source of stability, personal and financial fulfillment, the precariousness of work and frayed interpersonal relationships, which tend to induce suffering and illness, have been highlighted (LAGO; CUNHA; BORGES, 2015). This may have had a more pronounced effect on the biology and medicine teachers in this study. Thus, there is a need for reflection on the subject among teachers, educational institutions and society, with a view to promoting a better quality of life for this public (FERREIRA *et al.*, 2015; LAGO; CUNHA; BORGES, 2015).

CONCLUSION

The good quality of life found in most of the domains could provide positive moments for the health teachers at this institution. However, as the teachers who took part in this study had a regular quality of life in the physical domain, this aspect requires attention, since the association of a good quality of life in all the domains influences a better quality of life in general.

The associations between sociodemographic and academic characteristics and quality of life showed that teachers who have been working for more than 12 years, who do not have a partner, who do not live with their families and who are under 43 years of age need more care, highlighting the need for intervention for these workers. Special attention is needed for biology and medicine teachers, whose quality of life was most affected.

It is worth highlighting the need to investigate this issue with a view to improving the daily lives and work of teachers. It is therefore recommended that further research be carried out in the context of this study and in other higher education institutions. It is hoped that this study will help higher education institutions to take effective action in the field of health promotion and in promoting advances in the quality of life of university teachers.

REFERENCES

ALMEIDA, B.A.M.; GUITIERREZ, L.G.; MARQUES R. **Quality of life:** definition, concepts and interfaces with other areas of research. Sao Paulo: School of Arts, Sciences and Humanities, 2012.

ALVES, J. G. B.; TENÓRIO, M.; ANJOS, A. G. dos; FIGUEROA, J. N. Quality of life in medical students at the beginning and end of the course: evaluation by Whoqol-bref. **Revista Brasileira de Educaçâo Mèdica**, v. 34, n. 1, p. 91-96, jan./mar. 2010.

ARRONQUI, G.V.; LACAVA, R.M.V.B.; MAGALHÂES, S.M.F.; GOLDMAN, R.E. Perceptions of nursing students on their quality of life. **Acta Paulista de Enfermagem**, v.24, n.6, p.762-765, 2011.

BARROS, A. de J. P. de B.; LEHFELD, N. A. de S. **Projeto de Pesquisa:** Propostas Metodológicas. 18. ed. Petrópolis, Rio de Janeiro: Vozes, 2009. 321 p.

BECK, C. L. C.; BUDÓ, M. de L. D.; GONZALES, R. M. B. A qualidade de vida na concepção de um grupo de professores de enfermagem - elementos para reflexao. **Revista da Escola de Enfermagem da Universidade de Sâo Paulo**, Sao Paulo, v. 33, n. 4, p. 348-354, dec. 1999.

BOWLING, A. **Measuring health***:* a review of quality of life measurement scales. 2. ed. Buckingham: Open University Press, 1997. 159 p.

BRAZIL. Ministry of Health. **Work-related illnesses**. Manual of Procedures for Health Services. Brasilia (DF): Ministry of Health, 2001. 580 p. (Series A. Normas e Manuais Técnicos; n.114).

CAMPONOGARA, S.; KIRCHHOF, A. L. C.; RAMOS, F. R. S. Perspectives for quality of life and health promotion in the context of the risk society. **Ciência, Cuidado e Saùde**, Maringa, v. 7, n. 4, p. 551-557, Oct./Dec. 2008.

CARAN, V. C. S.; FREITAS, F. C. T. de; ALVES, L. A.; PEDRÂO, L. J.; ROBAZZI, M. L. do C. C. Psychosocial occupational risks and their repercussions on the health of university teachers. **Revista Enfermagem Universidade Estadual do Rio de Janeiro**, Rio de Janeiro, v. 19, n. 2, p. 255-261, Apr./Jun. 2011.

CARR, A. J.; GIBSON, B.; ROBSON, P. G. Is quality of life determined by expectations or experience? **Helping doctors make better decisions**, v. 322, n. 322, p. 1240-1243, 2001.

CASTELLANOS, P. L. **Epidemiology, public health, health status and living conditions:** conceptual considerations. In: BARATA, R. B. Condiçoes de vida e situaçâo de saù saúde. Rio de Janeiro: ABRASCO, p. 31-75, 1997 (ABRASCO. Saùde Movimento, 4).

CONCEIÇÂO, M. R. da.; ALVES, M. D. S.; COSTA, M. S.; ALMEIDA, M. I. de.; ALVES E SOUZA, A. M.; CAVALCANTE, M. B. de. P. T. Qualidade de vida do enfermeiro no trabalho docente: estudo com o *WHOQOL-bref.* **Escola de Enfermagem Anna Nery**, Rio de Janeiro, v. 16, n. 2, p. 320-325, abr./jun. 2012.

COSTA, M. A. F.; COSTA, M. de F. B. **Projeto** de **Pesquisa:** entenda e faz. Petrópolis, Rio de Janeiro: Vozes, 2012. 140 p.

CRESWELL, J. W. **Research design:** qualitative, quantitative and mixed methods. 3. ed. Porto Alegre: Artmed, 2010. 296 p.

COGO, L.L.R.; GONÇALVES, L.O.; KERKOSKI, E.; SANTOS, A.A.; CHESANI, F.H. Perfil da qualidade de vida dos fisioterapeutas docentes do curso de fisioterapia da Universidade do Vale do Itajai. **Revista Contexto Saùde**, v. 20, n. 10, p. 367-74, 2011.

DAVILA, M.H.X.; CASAGRANDE, R.J.T.; PEREIRA, V.C.G. Qualidade de vida do trabalhador de uma instituição de ensino. **Caderno Saùde Pùblica**, v. 4, n. 1, p. 110-26, 2010.

DAMASIO, B.F.; MELO, R.L.P.; SILVA, J.P. Sense of life, psychological well-being and quality of life in school teachers. **Paidéia**, v. 54, n. 23, p. 73-82, 2013.

FARQUHAR, M. Definitions of quality of life: a taxonomy. **Journal of Advanced Nursing**, v. 22, p. 502-508, 1995.

FERNANDES, M.H.; ROCHA, V.M.; FAGUNDES, A.A.R. Impacto da sintomatologia osteomuscular na qualidade de vida de professores. **Revista Brasileira**

de Epidemiologia, v. 14, n. 2, p. 276-84, 2011.

FERREIRA, R.C.; SILVEIRA, A.P.; BARBOSA DE SA, M.A.; FERES, S.B.L.; SOUZA, J.G.S.; MARTINS, A.M.E.B.L. Mental disorder and stressors at work among university professors in the health area. **Revista Trabalho Educaçâo e Saùde**, v.13, supl. 1, p. 135-55, 2015.

FERREIRA, E. M.; FERNANDES, M. F. P.; PRADO, C.; BAPTISTA, P. C. P.; FREITAS, G. F.; BONINI, B. B. Prazer e sofrimento no processo de trabalho do enfermeiro docente. **Revista Escola de Enfermagem da Universidade de Sao Paulo**, Sao Paulo, v. 43, n. 2, p. 1292-1296, 2009.

FIEDLER, P. T. **Evaluation of the quality of life of medical students and the influence exerted by academic training.** 2008. 266 f. Thesis (Doctorate in Sciences) - Faculty of Medicine, University of Sao Paulo, Sao Paulo, 2008.

FILHO, A.O.; NETTO-OLIVEIRA, E.R.; OLIVEIRA, A.A.B. Quality of life and risk factors of university professors. **Revista da Educaçâo Fisica/UEM**, v. 23, n. 1, p. 57-67, 2012.

FLECK, M. P. A.; LOUZADA, S.; XAVIER, M.; CHACHAMOVICH, E.; VIEIRA, G.; SANTOS, L.; PINZON, V. Aplicação da versão em português do instrumento abreviado de avaliaçâo da qualidade de vida "WHOQOL-Bref". **Revista de Saùde Pùblica**, Sao Paulo, v. 34, n. 2, p. 178-183, abr. 2000.

FLECK, M. P. A.; LOUZADA, S.; XAVIER, M.; CHACHAMOVICH, E.; VIEIRA, G.; SANTOS, L.; PINZON, V. Application of the Portuguese version of the World Health Organization's quality of life instrument (WHOQOL-100). **Revista de Saùde Pùblica**, Sao Paulo, v. 33, n. 2, p. 198-205, abr. 1999.

GAMPEL, D.; KARSCH, U. M.; FERREIRA, L. P. Voice perception and quality of life in elderly teachers and non-teachers. **Ciência & Saùde Coletiva**, Rio de Janeiro, v. 15, n. 6, p. 2907-2916, 2010.

GARCIA, A.L.; OLIVEIRA, E.R.A.; BARROS, E.B. Qualidade de vida de professores do ensino superior na área da saúde: discurso e pràtica cotidiana. **Cogitare**

Enfermagem, v. 13, n.1, p. 18-24, jan./mar. 2008.

GIL, A. C. **Como elaborar Projetos de Pesquisa.** 5. ed. Sao Paulo: Atlas, 2010. 184 p.

KOETZ, L.; REMPEL, C.; PÉRICO, E. Quality of life of teachers at community higher education institutions in Rio Grande do Sul. **Revista Ciência & Saùde Coletiva,** v. 18, n. 4, p. 1019-28, 2013.

KOIFMAN, L. The role of the university and medical education. **Revista Brasileira de Educaçâo Mèdica**, Rio de Janeiro, v. 35, n. 2, p. 145-146, Apr./Jun. 2011.

KLUTHCOVSKY, A. C.G. C; KLUTHCOVSKY, F.A. The WHOQOL-bref, an instrument for assessing quality of life: a systematic review. **Revista de Psiquiatria** do Rio Grande do Sul, Rio Grande do Sul, v. 3, n. 3, 2009.

LAGO, R.R.; CUNHA, B.S.; BORGES, M.F.S.O. Perception of teaching work at a university in the northern region of Brazil. **Revista Trabalho Educaçâo e Saùde,** v. 13, n. 2, p. 429-50, 2015.

MARCOS, B. Ethics **and Health Professionals.** Sao Paulo: Santos livraria e editora, 1999. 238 p.

MARTINEZ, K. A. S. C.; VITTA, A.; LOPES, E. S. Avaliação da qualidade de vida dos professores universitârios da cidade de Bauru-SP. **Salusvita,** Bauru, v. 28, n. 3, p. 217224, 2009.

MEDEIROS, J. B. **Redaçâo Cientifica:** a pràtica de fichamentos, resumos, resenhas. 11. ed. Sao Paulo: Atlas, 2009. 336 p.

MINAYO, M. C. de S.; HARTZ, Z. M. de A.; BUSS, P. M. Qualidade de vida e saùde: um debate necessàrio. **Ciência e Saùde Coletiva**, Rio de Janeiro, v. 5, n. 1, p. 7-18, 2000.

MORAIS, E.P.G.; AZEVEDO, R.R.; CHIARI, B.M. Correlation between voice, vocal self-assessment and voice quality of life in female teachers. **Revista CEFAC,** v. 14, n. 5, p. 892-900, 2012.

MULATO, S. C.; BUENO, S. M. V.; FRANCO, D. M. Teaching in Nursing: dissatisfactions and unfavorable indicators. **Acta Paulista de Enfermagem,** Sao Paulo, v. 23, n. 6, p. 769-774, 2010.

OLIVEIRA, R. A.; CIAMPONE, M. H. T. Quality of life of nursing students: the construction of a process and interventions. **Revista Escola de Enfermagem da Universidade de Sao Paulo,** Sao Paulo, v. 42, n. 1, p. 57-65, 2008.

OLIVEIRA, B. M.; MININEL, V. A.; FELLI, V. E. A. Quality of life of undergraduate nursing students. **Revista Brasileira de Enfermagem,** Brasilia, v. 64, n. 1, p. 130-135, jan./feb. 2011.

OLIVEIRA; E. R. A. de.; GARCIA, A. L.; GOMES, M. J.; BITTAR, T. O.; PEREIRA, A. C. Gender and perceived quality of life - a study with health professors. **Ciência & Saùde Coletiva**, Rio de Janeiro, v. 17, n. 3, p. 741-747, mar. 2012.

PANZINI, R. G.; ROCHA, N. S. da; BANDEIRA, D. R.; FLECK, M. P. de A. Qualidade de vida e espiritualidade. **Revista de Psiquiatria Clinica,** Sao Paulo, v. 34, supl. 1, p. 105-115, 2007.

PASCHOAL, S. M. P. **Quality of life in the elderly:** development of an instrument that privileges their opinion. 2001. Master's dissertation - Faculty of Medicine, University of Sao Paulo, Sao Paulo, 2001.

PENTEADO, R. Z.; PEREIRA, I. M. T. B. Quality of life and vocal health of teachers. **Revista de Saùde Pùblica,** Sao Paulo, v. 41, n. 2, p. 236-243, abr. 2007.

PEREIRA, E.F.; TEIXEIRA, C.S.; LOPES, A.D.S. Quality of life of elementary school teachers in the municipality of Florianópolis, SC, Brazil. **Journal Ciência & Saùde Coletiva,** v. 18, n. 7, p. 1963-70, 2013.

PETRINI, A.C. Evaluation of the perception of quality of life of young university students: comparison between day and night shift undergraduates. **Revista Brasileira de Qualidade de Vida,** v.5,n.3, p.1-8, 2013.

POLIT, D. F.; BECK, C. T.; HUNGLER, B. P. **Fundamentals of Nursing Research.** 7. ed. Porto Alegre: Artmed, 2011. 488 p.

RAMOS, F. R. S.; BORGES, L. M.; BREHMER, L. C. de F.; SILVEIRA, L. R. Ethical training of nurses - indications of change in the perception of teachers. **Acta Paulista de Enfermagem,** Sao Paulo, v. 24, n. 4, p. 485-492, 2011.

RAVAGNANI, L.M.B.; DOMINGOS, N.A.M.; MIYAZAKI, M. C. O. S. Quality of life and coping strategies in patients undergoing renal transplantation. **Estudos de Psicologia (Natal),** Natal, v.12, n. 2, p. 177-184, 2007.

ROCHA, S. S. L.; FELLI, V. E. A. Qualidade de vida no trabalho docente em enfermagem. **Revista Latino-Americana de Enfermagem**, Rio de Janeiro, v.12, n.1, p. 28-35, jan./feb. 2004.

SALLES, W.N.; EGERLAND, E.M.; BARROSO, M.L.C.; SOUZA, C.A. Lifestyle and socioeconomic profile of teachers of Physical Education courses at the Federal University of Santa Catarina - UFSC. **Revista Brasileira de Ciências da Saùde**, v. 34, n.10, p. 7-14, 2012.

SANTOS, I.; CAVALCANTE, L. B.; BERARDINELLI, L. M. M. Study on the life habits of nursing teachers according to Roy's adaptive modes. **Revista de Enfermagem UERJ**, Rio de Janeiro, v. 18, n. 1, p. 48-54, jan./marc. 2010.

SEIDL, E.M.F; ZANNON, C.M.L.C. Quality of life and health: conceptual and methodological aspects. **Cadernos de Saùde Pùblica**, Rio de Janeiro, v. 20, n. 2, p. 580-588, 2004.

SILVA, M.L.S.; ARPINI, D.M. The new national adoption law - challenges for family reintegration. **Psicologia em Estudo,** v. 18, n.1, p.125-35, 2013.

SILVÉRIO, M.R.; PATRiCIO, Z.M.; BRODBECK, I.M.; GROSSEMAN, S. Teaching in the health area and its repercussions on teachers' quality of life. **Revista Brasileira de Educaçâo Mèdica**, Rio de Janeiro, v. 34, n. 1, p. 65-73, 2010.

TERRA, F. de S.; SECCO, I. A. de O.; ROBAZZI, M. L. do C. C. Profile of teachers in undergraduate nursing courses at public and private universities. **Revista de Enfermagem UERJ**, Rio de Janeiro, v. 19, n. 1, p. 26-33, jan./mar. 2011.

VERGARA, S. C. **Methods of Data Collection in the Field**. Sâo Paulo: Atlas, 2009.

98 p.

WHOQOL GROUP. WHOQOL GROUP. **The development of the World Health Organization quality of life assessment instrument (the WHOQOL).**In ORLEY, J.; KUYKEN, W. (editors). Quality of life assessment: international perspectives. Heidelberg: Springer - Verlag;.p. 41-60, 1994.

WHOQOL GROUP. Development of the World Health Organization WHOQOL-Bref quality of life assessment. **PsycholMed,** v. 28, p. 551-558, 2000.

XAVIER, M. Trabalho e sonhos: desejos e pesadelos de professores e trabalhadores da saúde na era do capitalismo organizational. **Cadernos de Psicologia Social do Trabalho,** v. 14, n. 1, p. 93-110, 2011.

ZHAN, L. Qualityoflife: conceptual andmeasurementissues. **Journal Of Advanced Nursing,** v.17, p.795- 800, jul. 1992.

ANNEXES

ANNEX A

FREE AND INFORMED CONSENT TO PARTICIPATE IN RESEARCH

Title of the research: Quality of Life of Teachers of Undergraduate Courses at the Center for Biological and Health Sciences of a Public University in Minas Gerais **Promoting institution:** State University of Montes Claros.

Sponsor: Not applicable

Coordinator: Prof. Ms. Maria Aparecida Vieira.

Attention:

Before agreeing to take part in this research, it is important that you read and understand the following explanation of the proposed procedures. This statement describes the purpose, methodology/procedures, benefits, risks, discomforts and precautions of the study. It also describes the alternative procedures that are available to you and your right to withdraw from the study at any time. No guarantees or promises can be made about the results of the study.

1. Objective: To evaluate the quality of life of the teachers of the Undergraduate Courses in the Health Area of the State University of Montes Claros.

2. Methodology/procedures: This is a quantitative and descriptive study, whose subjects will be the teachers of the Undergraduate Courses in the Health Area of the State University of Montes Claros, Minas Gerais. Two instruments will be used to collect data: a generic questionnaire on quality of life from the World Health Organization, called the *World Health Organization's Abbreviated Quality of Life Assessment Tool* (WHOQOL-Bref), which consists of the abbreviated version of the WHOQOL-100, developed by the World Health Organization's Quality of Life Group, and another to collect complementary information, consisting of variables relating to the sociodemographic aspects of the involved in this study. Data collection will only be carried out after this project has been approved by the Research Ethics Committee of the State University of Montes Claros.

3. **Justification:** Considering that the university space can foster or not experiences that contribute to the quality of life of teaching professionals, it is important to carry out this research so that it can support, as a source of information, the elaboration of support and coping strategies for teachers in the health area; as well as the implementation of formalized spaces dedicated to their real realities, in order to generate learning opportunities that facilitate the resolution of difficult situations in their daily lives and in their profession.

4. **Benefits:** This research will make it possible to find out about the quality of life of health professors at UNIMONTES, the results of which could be used as a source of information to draw up support and coping strategies for professors in this area, as well as to set up formalized spaces dedicated to their real realities, in order to generate learning opportunities that facilitate the resolution of difficult situations in their daily lives and in their profession.

5. **Discomfort and risks:** No physical or moral discomfort or risks are anticipated.

6. **Damages:** No physical or moral damage is foreseen.

7. **Alternative methodology/procedures available:** Not applicable.

8. **Confidentiality of information:** The information provided will only be used for scientific purposes, and the participants in the research will have their identity preserved.

9. **Compensation/indemnity:** Since no risks, discomfort or moral or physical damage to the research participants are foreseen, no form of compensation or reward is foreseen either.

10. **Other relevant information:** not applicable.

11. **Consent: I** have read and understood the preceding information. I have had the opportunity to ask questions and all my doubts have been answered to my satisfaction. This form is being signed voluntarily by me, indicating my consent to participate in

this research, until I decide otherwise. I will receive a signed copy of this consent form. In the case of research to be carried out with minors, I will take responsibility for the disclosure of the data.

Participant's name	Participant's signature	Date
Participant's name	Participant's signature	Date
Name of witness	Participant's signature	Date
Prof. Maria Aparecida Vieira	Signature of Research Coordinator	Date

Name of Research Coordinator: Prof^a. Maria Aparecida Vieira

Researcher's address: Rua Jasmim, n° 127, Sagrada Familia CEP 39401-028 - Montes Claros - MG.

Phones: (38) 32122145 - Home.

(38) 32298285 - UNIMONTES Nursing Department.

ANNEX B

WHOQOL - ABBREVIATED

Portuguese version

MENTAL HEALTH PROGRAM

WORLD HEALTH ORGANIZATION

GENEVA

Coordination of the WHOQOL Group in Brazil

Dr. Marcelo Pio de Almeida Fleck

Adjunct Professor

Department of Psychiatry and Forensic Medicine Federal University of Rio Grande do Sul Porto Alegre - RS - Brazil

Instructions

This questionnaire is about how you feel about your quality of life, health and other areas of your life. **Please answer all the questions.** If you are not sure which answer to give to a question, please choose the one that seems most appropriate. This can often be your first choice.

Please bear in mind your values, aspirations, pleasures and concerns. We're asking you how you feel about your life, taking the **last two weeks** as a reference. For example, thinking about the last two weeks, a question could be:

	nothing	very little	medium	very	completely
Do you get the support you need from others?	I	2	3	4	5

You should circle the number that best corresponds to how much support you have received from others over the last two weeks. Therefore, you should circle number 4 if you received "milito" support as below.

	nothing	very little	medium	very	completely
Do you get the support you need from others?	1	2	3	4	5

You should circle number 1 if you have received "nothing" in support.

Please read each question, see what you think and circle the number and you'll find the best answer.

		very bad	Riim	neither Riim nor good	good	very good
1	How would you rate your quality of life?	1	2	3	4	5

		very dissatisfied	dissatisfied	Neither satisfied nor dissatisfied	Satisfied	very Satisfied
2	How satisfied are you with your health?	1	2	3	4	5

The following questions are about **how much** you've been feeling certain things over the last two weeks.

		nothing	very little	more or less	a lot	extremely
3	To what extent do you think your (physical) pain prevents you from doing what you need to do?	1	2	3	4	5
4	How much do you need medical treatment to go about your daily life?	1	2	3	4	5
5	How much do you enjoy life?	1	2	3	4	5
6	How meaningful do you think your life is?	1	2	3	4	5
7	How well can you concentrate?	1	2	3	4	5
8	How safe do you feel in your daily life?	1	2	3	4	5
9	How healthy is your physical environment (climate, noise, pollution, attractions)?	1	2	3	4	5

The following questions ask **how fully** you have felt or been able to do certain things in the last two weeks.

		nothing	very little	medium	very	completely

10	Do you have enough energy for your day-to-day life?	1	2	3	4	5
Il	Are you able to accept your physical appearance?	1	2	3	4	5
12	Do you have enough money to meet your needs?	1	2	3	4	5
13	How available is the information you need in your daily life?	1	2	3	4	5
14	To what extent do you have opportunities for leisure activities?	I	2	3	4	5

The following questions ask **how good or satisfied** you felt about various aspects of your life in the last two weeks.

		very me	reno	nor me nor boni	good	very good
15	How well can you move?	1	2	3	4	5

		very dissatisfied	unsatisfied	nor satisfied nor dissatisfied	satisfied	very satisfied
16	How satisfied are you with your sleep?	1	2	3	4	5
17	How satisfied are you with your ability to carry out your day-to-day activities?	1	2	3	4	5
1 8	How satisfied are you with your ability to work?	1	2	3	4	5
19	How satisfied are you with yourself?	1	2	3	4	5
20	How satisfied are you with your personal relationships (friends, relatives, acquaintances, colleagues)?	1	2	3	4	5
21	How satisfied are you with your sex life?	1	2	3	4	5
22	How satisfied are you with the support you receive from your friends?	1	2	3	4	5
23	How satisfied are you with the conditions where you live?	1	2	3	4	5
24	How satisfied are you with your access to health services?	1	2	3	4	5

25	How satisfied are you with your means of transport?	1	2	3	4	5

The following questions refer to **how often** you have felt or experienced certain things in the last two weeks.

		never	sometimes	Frequency -of course	very frequently	always
26	How often do you experience negative feelings such as bad moods, despair, anxiety or depression?	I	2	3	4	5

Did anyone help you fill in this questionnaire?...

How long did it take you to fill in this questionnaire? ....

Do you have any comments on the questionnaire?

THANK YOU FOR YOUR COOPERATION

ANNEX C

INSTITUTION'S AGREEMENT TO PARTICIPATE IN RESEARCH IN RESEARCH

Title of the study: Quality of Life of Teachers of Undergraduate Courses at the Center for Biological and Health Sciences of a Public University in Minas Gerais

Institution where the research will be carried out: State University of Montes Claros

Researcher responsible: Prof. Ms. Maria Aparecida Vieira

Address and telephone number: Rua Jasmim, n° 127, Bairro Sagrada Familia, CEP 39401-028 - Montes Claros - MG.

Phones: (38) 3212-2145 Residence

(38) 3229-8285 Department of Nursing, UNIMONTES.

Attention:

Before agreeing to take part in this research, it is important that you read and understand the following explanation of the proposed procedures. This statement describes the purpose, methodology/procedures, benefits, risks, discomforts and precautions of the study. It also describes the alternative procedures that are available to you and your right to withdraw from the study at any time. No guarantees or promises can be made about the results of the study.

1. Objective: To evaluate the quality of life of the teachers of the Undergraduate Courses in the Health Area of the State University of Montes Claros.

2. Methodology/procedures: This is a quantitative and descriptive study, whose subjects will be the teachers of the Undergraduate Courses in the Health Area of the State University of Montes Claros, Minas Gerais. Data will be collected using the World Health Organization's generic questionnaire on quality of life, called the *World* Health *Organization's Abbreviated Quality of Life Assessment Tool* (WHOQOL-Bref), which consists of the abbreviated version of the WHOQOL-100, developed by the World Health Organization's Quality of Life Group, and another to collect complementary information, consisting of variables relating to the socio-demographic aspects of those involved in this study. Data collection will only take place after this project has been approved by the Research Ethics Committee of the State University of Montes Claros.

3. Justification: Considering that the space at the university may or may not foster experiences that contribute to the quality of life of these teachers, it is important to carry out this research so that it can subsidize, as a source of information, the elaboration of support and coping strategies for teachers in the health area; as well as the implementation of formalized spaces dedicated to their real realities, in order to generate learning opportunities that facilitate the resolution of difficult situations in their daily lives and in their profession.

4. Benefits: This research will make it possible to find out about the quality of life of UNIMONTES health professors, the results of which will be used as a source of information for the development of support and coping strategies for health professors, as well as the implementation of formalized spaces dedicated to their real realities, in order to generate learning opportunities that facilitate the resolution of difficult situations in their daily lives and in their profession.

5. Discomforts and risks: No physical or moral discomforts or risks are anticipated.

6. **Damages:** No physical or moral damage is foreseen.

7. **Alternative methodology/procedures available:** Not applicable.

8. **Confidentiality of information:** The information provided will only be used for scientific purposes, and the participants in the research will have their identity preserved.

9. **Compensation/indemnity:** Since no risks, discomfort or moral or physical damage to the research participants are foreseen, no form of compensation or reward is foreseen either.

10. **Other relevant information:** not applicable.

11. **Consent: I** have read and understood the preceding information. I have had the opportunity to ask questions and all my doubts have been answered to my satisfaction. This form is being signed voluntarily by me, indicating my consent to participate in this institution, until I decide otherwise. I will receive a signed copy of this consent. And that it can only be approved in this institution after approval by the Ethics Committee of the institution promoting the research.

Prof. Maria das Mercês Borém Correa Machado. Director of the Center for Biological and Health Sciences

___/___/___

Signature and stamp of the person responsible for the institution Date

Prof. Maria Aparecida Vieira - Researcher responsible for the research

___/___/___

Signature

Date

APPENDIX

APPENDIX A

Title: Quality of Life of the Teachers of the Undergraduate Courses of the Center of Biological and Health Sciences of a Public University in Minas Gerais

SOCIODEMOGRAPHIC QUESTIONNAIRE

Dear Teacher:

We kindly ask you to answer the following questions, which are relevant to this research, which aims to evaluate the Quality of Life of the Teachers of the Undergraduate Courses of the Center for Biological and Health Sciences of the State University of Montes Claros.

There is no right or wrong alternative.

Thank you very much for your valuable attention!

01- What is your gender?

a) Male.

b) Female.

02- How old were you on March 31, 2013?

a) 20 to 29 years old.

b) 30 to 39 years old.

c) 40 to 49 years old.

d) 50 to 59 years old.

e) 60 or more.

03- What is your marital status?

a) Single.

b) Married.

c) Viùvo (a).

d) Legally separated or divorced.

e) Another situation.

04- You consider yourself:

a) White (a).

b) Black.

c) Brown.

d) Indigenous.

e) Oriental.

f) Undeclared.

05- Where were you born?

a) In Montes Claros.

b) In another town in the north of Minas Gerais.

c) In a city in another region of Minas Gerais.

d) In a city in another state.

e) Abroad.

06- Where do you currently live?

a) In the city of Montes Claros.

b) In another town in the north of Minas Gerais.

c) In a city in the northwest of Minas /Vale do Mucuri or Jequitinhonha.

d) In a city in the state of Bahia.

e) In a city in another state.

f) In another country.

07- You live:

a) With his own family.

b) With relatives.

c) Alone.

d) Another situation.

08- Do you have another job besides teaching at the State University of Montes Claros?

a) No.

b) Teaching at another Higher Education Institution.

c) Teaching at other Higher Education Institutions.

d) Teaching at another educational institution.

e) Primary Health Care.

f) Hospital Care.

g) Management Positions, Consulting.

h) Other.

09- How long have you been teaching in higher education?

a) Up to 09 years old.

b) Between 10 and 19 years old.

c) Between 20 and 29 years old.

c) Over 30 years old.

10- What is your employment relationship with the department of the course you teach at the State University of Montes Claros?

a) Hired/Designated.

b) Effective.

c) Exclusive Dedication.

d) Extended Day.

11- You did your undergraduate degree:

a) All at a public higher education institution.

b) All at a private higher education institution.

c) Mostly in a public higher education institution.

d) Mostly in private higher education institutions.

e) Another situation.

12- How involved are you in the economic life of your family group?

a) I work and am only responsible for my own livelihood.

b) I work and I'm responsible for my livelihood and I partly contribute to supporting my family.

c) I work and I'm the main breadwinner.

13- In which range does the gross monthly income (without discounts) of your family group best fit (sum of your income, that of your parents, siblings, spouse, children, etc.)?

a) Between R$ 622.00 and R$ 1,866.00.

b) Between R$1,867.00 and R$3,110.00.

c) Between R$ 3,111.00 and R$ 4,354.00.

d) Between R$ 4,355.00 and R$ 6,220.00.

e) Between R$ 6,221.00 and R$ 12,440.00.

f) Above R$ 12,440.00.

14- What is your schooling?

a) Complete university degree. What course did you take? (please list the main one)

b) *Lato sensu* postgraduate course - Specialization - in progress.

c) *Lato sensu* postgraduate course - Specialization - complete.

d) *Stricto sensu* postgraduate course - Master's degree in progress.

e) *Stricto sensu* postgraduate degree - Master's degree completed.

f) *Stricto sensu* postgraduate studies - Doctorate in progress.

g) *Stricto sensu* postgraduate degree - Doctorate completed.

h) Post-doctorate in progress.

i) Post-doctorate completed.

15- Apart from academic books, how many books do you read a year?

a) None.

b) 01 to 02 books.

c) 03 to 05 books.

d) More than 5 books.

16- Cigarettes are proven to be harmful to health. Where do you stand?

a) I don't smoke.

b) Smoke.

17- Do you have a computer at home?

a) No.

b) Yes, with internet access.

c) Yes, without internet access.

18- What is your main source of information about current events?

a) Written newspaper.

b) News.

c) Radio news.

d) Magazines.

e) Internet.

f) Another source.

g) I don't keep up to date.

19- Which of the activities listed below do you spend the most time on, apart from teaching?

a) Watching TV.

b) Going to the theater/cinema.

c) Listening to music.

d) Going to bars, nightclubs, etc.

e) Reading.

20- What is your religion?

a) Catholic.

b) Evangelical.

c) Adventist.

d) Other.

e) None.

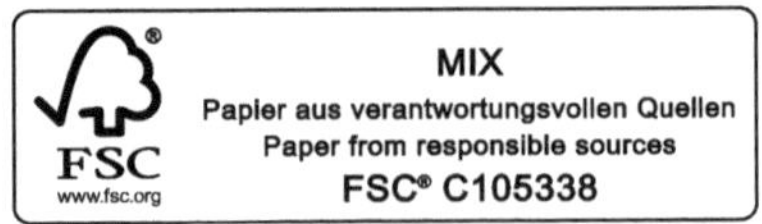

Printed by Books on Demand GmbH, Norderstedt / Germany